Acid Reflux Diet Cookbook For Seniors

Discover Delicious, Easy-to-Prepare Meals and Snacks Specially Designed for Older Adults, with Budget-Friendly Options and Heartburn-Relieving Strategies

Dr. Juliana Andrew

Copyright © 2024 by Dr. Juliana Andrew

All rights reserved. No part of this book may be reproduced in any form or by any electronic or mechanical means, including information storage and retrieval systems, without permission in writing from the publisher, except by a reviewer who may quote brief passages in a Review.

The information provided in this book is for educational purposes and is not intended as a substitute for professional medical advice, diagnosis, or treatment. Always seek the advice of your physician or other qualified health provider with any questions you may have regarding a medical condition.

Table of Contents

Introduction: Reclaiming Joy at the Dinner Table 7

Chapter 1 11

    Understanding Acid Reflux in Seniors 11

    The Benefits of a Thoughtful Diet 12

    How to Use This Book 13

Chapter 2: Heartburn-Relieving Strategies 15

    Dietary Guidelines for Managing Acid Reflux 15

    Identifying and Avoiding Trigger Foods 16

    Meal Planning and Portion Control 19

    Lifestyle Modifications for Better Digestion 20

Chapter 3: Breakfast Delights 21

    Smoothie 21

    Recipe 1: Berry Blast 21

        Recipe 2: Creamy Avocado Spinach Smoothie 22

        Recipe 3: Banana Almond Butter Smoothie 23

        Recipe 4: Simple Oatmeal with Apples and 24

        Recipe 5: Vegetable Omelette 25

        Recipe 6: Baked Oatmeal Cups 27

        Recipe 7: Quinoa Breakfast Bowl 29

        Recipe 8: Creamy Coconut Chia Pudding 30

        Recipe 9: Classic Peanut Butter Toast 31

        Recipe 10: Apple Cinnamon Baked Oatmeal 32

        Recipe 11: Spinach and Feta Omelette 33

        Recipe 12: Blueberry Almond Smoothie Bowl 35

Recipe 13: Apple Cinnamon Breakfast Quinoa 36

Recipe 14: Peanut Butter Banana Breakfast 37

Recipe 15: Chia Seed Breakfast Pudding 38

Chapter 4 39

   Soothing Soups and Salads 39

      Recipe 1: Chicken and Vegetable Broth Soup 39

      Recipe 2: Lentil and Vegetable Soup 41

      Recipe 3: Creamy Butternut Squash Soup 43

      Recipe 4: Creamy Cauliflower Soup 44

      Recipe 5: Tomato and Basil Salad 45

      Recipe 6: Greek Salad 46

      Recipe 7: Avocado and Chickpea Salad 47

      Recipe 8: Roasted Vegetable Salad 49

      Recipe 9: Quinoa and Kale Salad 51

      Recipe 10: Spinach and Strawberry Salad 52

      Recipe 11: Creamy Carrot Ginger Soup 54

      Recipe 12: Creamy Mushroom Soup 56

      Recipe 13: Cucumber Tomato Salad 58

      Recipe 14: Spinach and Quinoa Salad 59

      Recipe 15: Watermelon Feta Salad 60

Chapter 5 61

   Main Course Meals 61

      Recipe 1: Lemon Herb Roasted Chicken 61

      Recipe 2: Garlic Butter Shrimp 61

      Recipe 3: Quinoa Stuffed Bell Peppers 63

      Recipe 4: Lentil and Vegetable Stir-Fry 65

Recipe 5: Slow-Cooker Vegetable Soup 66

Recipe 6: Turkey and Vegetable Stir-Fry 66

Recipe 7: Lemon Garlic Herb Tilapia........................ 68

Recipe 9: Coconut Curry Shrimp............................. 71

Recipe 10: Vegetarian Chili..................................... 72

Recipe 11: Herb-Roasted Turkey Breast.................. 74

Recipe 12: Lemon Garlic Shrimp Scampi................. 75

Recipe 13: Lentil Shepherd's Pie 76

Recipe 14: Vegetarian Lasagna............................... 78

Recipe 15: Slow-Cooker Vegetable Curry................ 80

Chapter 6 82

  Sides and Snacks.. 82

    Recipe 1: Garlic Herb Roasted Potatoes................. 82

    Recipe 2: Homemade Guacamole 83

    Recipe 3: Baked Zucchini Fries............................... 84

    Recipe 4: Cucumber Hummus Bites 86

    Recipe 5: Mini Oatmeal Banana Muffins 87

    Recipe 6: Roasted Cauliflower with Herbs 89

    Recipe 7: Creamy Spinach Dip 90

    Recipe 8: Quinoa Stuffed Bell Peppers 91

    Recipe 9: Baked Sweet Potato Fries....................... 93

    Recipe 10: Almond Butter Energy Balls 94

Chapter 7 95

  : Beverages and Desserts 95

    Recipe 1: Peppermint Tea 95

    Recipe 2: Ginger Turmeric Tea 96

Recipe 3: Honey Lemon Chamomile Tea 97

Recipe 4: Berry Smoothie 98

Recipe 5: Banana Oat Cookies 99

Recipe 6: Coconut Chia Pudding 100

Recipe 7: Apple Cinnamon Baked Oatmeal 101

Recipe 8: Avocado Chocolate Mousse 102

Recipe 9: Greek Yogurt Parfait 103

Recipe 10: Baked Apples with Cinnamon 104

Conclusion: A Toast to a Life Well-Lived, One Bite at a Time 105

Thanks for Reading 109

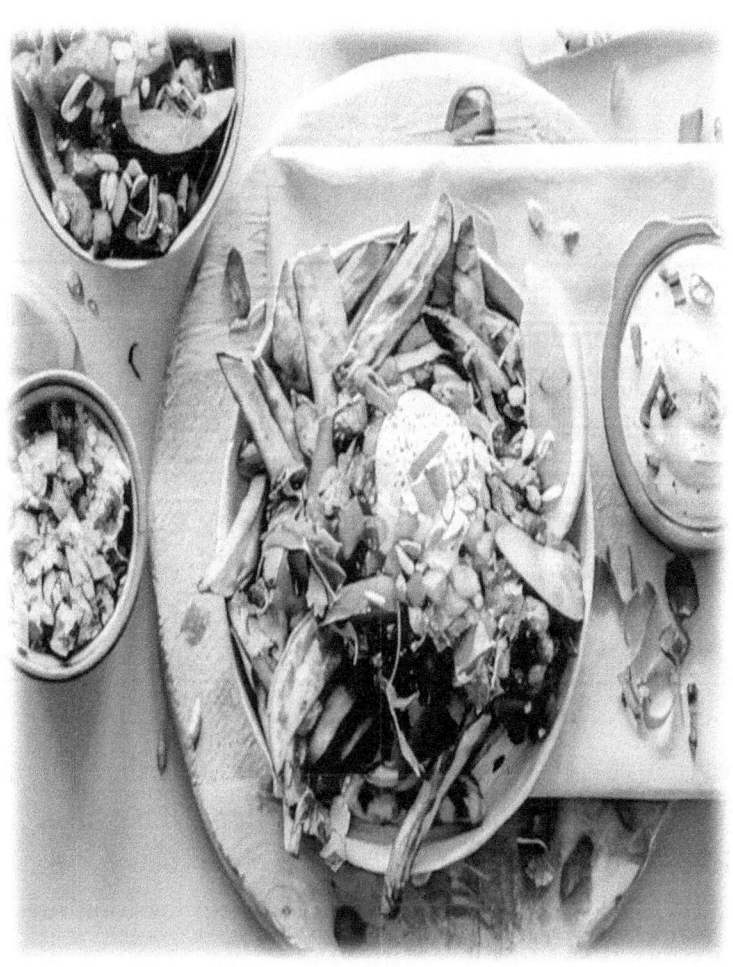

Introduction: Reclaiming Joy at the Dinner Table

Emily's heart sank as she felt the familiar burn of acid reflux creeping up her throat, a constant reminder of the discomfort that had become her unwelcome companion in recent years. What should have been a simple pleasure – enjoying a home-cooked meal with her family – was now overshadowed by the fear of triggering another painful episode.

For too long, Emily had resigned herself to a life of restrictive diets and avoiding her favorite dishes, all in an effort to keep the persistent heartburn at bay. But deep down, she longed for a sense of normalcy, a time when she could relish every bite without the looming threat of discomfort.

It was during a routine visit with her doctor that Emily's journey towards reclaiming her joy at the dinner table began. Her physician, recognizing the profound impact acid reflux had on Emily's quality of life, recommended a comprehensive approach that combined dietary modifications with lifestyle changes tailored specifically for older adults.

With a glimmer of hope, Emily embarked on this new path, armed with a wealth of knowledge and practical strategies. Step by step, she discovered the power of identifying and eliminating trigger foods, embracing heartburn-relieving alternatives, and implementing simple yet effective techniques to optimize her digestion.

As the weeks passed, Emily noticed a remarkable transformation. The once-dreaded mealtimes became occasions to savor, as she indulged in delicious, easy-to-prepare dishes that not only satisfied her taste buds but also provided lasting relief from acid reflux.

The budget-friendly recipes in this book became her trusted allies, proving that managing acid reflux didn't have to mean sacrificing flavor or breaking the bank. Each meal was a celebration of her renewed freedom, a testament to the power of knowledge and a thoughtful approach to self-care.

Emily's journey is a reminder that acid reflux, while challenging, is not an insurmountable obstacle. With the right guidance and a commitment to making positive changes, it is possible to reclaim the joy of dining, savoring every bite without the burden of discomfort.

If you, too, have found yourself longing for a life free from the grip of acid reflux, know that you are not alone. This book is your gateway to a world of possibilities, where delicious and heartburn-relieving meals become the norm, and the fear of discomfort fades into a distant memory.

Embark on your own transformative journey, secure in the knowledge that the path ahead is paved with practical solutions, heartwarming recipes, and the unwavering support of experts who understand the unique challenges faced by older adults. Rediscover the pure pleasure of shared meals, laughter, and cherished moments around the table – a life well-lived, one bite at a time.

Chapter 1

Embarking on a journey towards an acid reflux-free lifestyle is a transformative experience that promises to restore your vitality and zest for life. As we navigate the golden years, our bodies undergo natural changes that can make us more susceptible to the discomfort of acid reflux. However, by understanding the underlying causes and implementing thoughtful dietary and lifestyle adjustments, you can reclaim control and rediscover the joys of savoring every meal without the burden of heartburn.

In this comprehensive guide, we delve into the intricacies of acid reflux, arming you with the knowledge and practical strategies to effectively manage and alleviate your symptoms. Our approach is holistic, recognizing that a multifaceted approach is essential for long-lasting relief,

UNDERSTANDING ACID REFLUX IN SENIORS

Acid reflux, also known as gastroesophageal reflux disease (GERD), is a condition characterized by the backflow of stomach contents into the esophagus, causing a burning sensation in the chest and throat. As we age, factors such as weakened muscle tone, increased abdominal pressure, and changes in digestive enzymes can contribute to the development or exacerbation of acid reflux.

It's crucial to recognize that acid reflux is not an inevitable consequence of aging; rather, it is a condition that can be managed and mitigated through proactive measures. By gaining a deeper understanding of the underlying mechanisms and risk factors, you'll be better equipped to make informed choices that support your overall well-being.

THE BENEFITS OF A THOUGHTFUL DIET

One of the most powerful tools in managing acid reflux lies in the foods we consume. A carefully curated diet can not only alleviate symptoms but also promote healing and long-term relief. In this book, we'll guide you through the process of identifying and eliminating trigger foods that can exacerbate your condition, while introducing a wealth of delicious and nutrient-dense alternatives.

From alkaline-forming foods that neutralize stomach acid to fiber-rich options that promote healthy digestion, we'll explore a wide range of culinary delights that cater to your specific needs. By embracing a diet tailored to your individual circumstances, you'll experience a newfound freedom and joy in eating, without the fear of discomfort or pain.

How to Use This Book

This comprehensive guide is designed to be your steadfast companion on the journey towards an acid reflux-free lifestyle. Within its pages, you'll find a wealth of information, practical tips, and delectable recipes that seamlessly integrate into your daily routine.

We've structured the book in a logical and intuitive manner, ensuring that you can easily navigate through the various sections and find the specific guidance you need. Whether you're seeking insights on dietary modifications, stress management techniques, or exercise recommendations, this book will be your trusted source of knowledge.

.Embrace this book as a comprehensive resource, a trusted ally, and a source of empowerment. With dedication and the guidance provided within these pages, you'll unlock the key to a life free from the discomfort of acid reflux, enabling you to savor every moment and every meal with renewed vitality and joy.

Chapter 2: Heartburn-Relieving Strategies

In the quest for relief from the discomfort of acid reflux, knowledge is your most powerful ally. By understanding the intricate relationship between dietary choices, lifestyle habits, and heartburn, you can take control and implement effective strategies to alleviate your symptoms. This chapter will equip you with a comprehensive toolkit, empowering you to make informed decisions that promote lasting relief and overall well-being.

DIETARY GUIDELINES FOR MANAGING ACID REFLUX

The adage "you are what you eat" holds profound truth, especially when it comes to managing acid reflux. Certain foods can either soothe or exacerbate your condition, making it crucial to approach your diet with mindfulness and care. In this section, we'll provide you with heartburn-friendly and heartburn-triggering foods.

Embrace the power of alkaline-forming foods, which work in harmony with your body to neutralize excess stomach acid and promote a balanced digestive environment. From leafy greens and root vegetables to low-acid fruits and whole grains, you'll discover a world of nourishing options that not only taste delicious but also offer profound healing benefits.

IDENTIFYING AND AVOIDING TRIGGER FOODS

While general dietary guidelines provide a valuable foundation, it's essential to recognize that each individual's body may react differently to certain foods.

The foundation of managing acid reflux lies in dietary modifications. Here are some key principles to keep in mind:

Say "No" to Acidic Culprits: Certain foods can exacerbate acid production in your stomach. Common offenders include:

Citrus fruits (oranges, grapefruits)

Tomatoes (including tomato sauce, ketchup)

Spicy dishes (chili peppers, hot sauce)

Chocolate (especially dark chocolate)

Peppermint (including peppermint tea)

Fatty foods (fried foods, processed meats)

Carbonated beverages (soda, sparkling water)

Coffee (for some individuals)

Alcohol (can weaken the lower esophageal sphincter)

Embrace the Power of Alkaline Allies: Fruits and vegetables that lean towards the alkaline side of the pH scale can help neutralize stomach acid and provide soothing relief. Think about incorporating these into your meals:

Leafy greens (spinach, kale)

Melons (honeydew, cantaloupe)

Bananas

Root vegetables (potatoes, carrots)

Green beans

Cauliflower

Non-citrus fruits (apples, pears)

Spice it Up (Carefully): Spicy foods are notorious triggers for acid reflux. However, some herbs and spices can actually aid digestion. Experiment with these flavorful options:

Ginger

Turmeric

Fennel seed

Cumin

A sprinkle of cinnamon

Smaller, More Frequent Meals: Overeating stretches the stomach, putting pressure on the lower esophageal sphincter. Opt for smaller portions spread throughout the day to avoid overloading your digestive system.

MEAL PLANNING AND PORTION CONTROL

Planning your meals ahead of time can be a game-changer, especially when managing acid reflux. Here are some tips to get you started:

Plan Weekly Menus: Dedicate some time each week to plan your meals. This reduces stress around mealtimes and ensures you have heartburn-friendly options readily available.

Embrace Batch Cooking: Cook larger portions of protein sources like chicken or fish on the weekends. This allows you to easily whip up healthy meals throughout the week without spending extra time in the kitchen.

Portion Perfection: Use smaller plates and bowls to visually limit portion sizes and prevent overeating.

Focus on Nutrient Density: Prioritize foods rich in vitamins, minerals, and fiber to support overall gut health and aid digestion. Think colorful vegetables, whole grains, and lean protein sources.

Lifestyle Modifications for Better Digestion

While dietary changes are crucial, managing acid reflux is a holistic endeavor. Here are some lifestyle modifications that can significantly improve digestion and reduce heartburn:

- **Gravity is Your Friend:** Elevate the head of your bed by 6-8 inches using pillows or bed wedges. This keeps stomach acid from traveling back up the esophagus while you sleep.

- **Chew, Chew, Chew:** Proper chewing breaks down food, making it easier to digest and reducing strain on your digestive system.

- **Manage Stress:** Stress can exacerbate acid reflux. Explore relaxation techniques like yoga, meditation, or deep breathing to combat stress and promote gut health.

- **Loose the Tight Fit:** Tight-fitting clothing around the waist can put pressure on your stomach, increasing the risk of acid reflux. Opt for looser-fitting clothing to allow for comfortable digestion.

- **Listen to Your Body:** Pay attention to how your body reacts after meals. Avoid strenuous activity within 2-3 hours after eating to allow for proper digestion.

Chapter 3: Breakfast Delights

SMOOTHIE

RECIPE 1: BERRY BLAST

INGREDIENTS:

- 1/2 cup mixed berries (strawberries, blueberries, raspberries)
- 1/2 banana
- 1/2 cup Greek yogurt (unsweetened)
- 1/4 cup almond milk (unsweetened)
- 1 tablespoon honey (optional)

Instructions:

1. Wash the berries.
2. Peel and slice the banana.
3. In a blender, combine berries, banana, Greek yogurt, almond milk, and honey.
4. Blend until smooth.
5. Pour into a glass and enjoy this refreshing smoothie.

Recipe 2: Creamy Avocado Spinach Smoothie

Ingredients:

- 1/2 avocado
- 1 cup spinach leaves
- 1/2 cup pineapple chunks
- 1/2 cup coconut water (unsweetened)
- 1 tablespoon lemon juice

Instructions:

1. Peel and pit the avocado.
2. Wash the spinach leaves.
3. In a blender, combine avocado, spinach, pineapple chunks, coconut water, and lemon juice.
4. Blend until smooth.
5. Pour into a glass and savor the creamy texture of this nutritious smoothie.

Recipe 3: Banana Almond Butter Smoothie

Ingredients:

- 1 banana
- 2 tablespoons almond butter
- 1 cup almond milk (unsweetened)
- 1/2 teaspoon cinnamon
- Ice cubes

Instructions:

1. Peel and slice the banana.
2. In a blender, combine banana slices, almond butter, almond milk, cinnamon, and ice cubes.
3. Blend until smooth.
4. Pour into a glass and enjoy this protein-rich smoothie.

Recipe 4: Simple Oatmeal with Apples and Cinnamon

Ingredients:

- 1/2 cup rolled oats
- 1 cup water or milk of choice
- 1/2 apple, diced
- 1/2 teaspoon cinnamon
- 1 tablespoon honey (optional)

Instructions:

1. In a small saucepan, bring water or milk to a boil.

2. Stir in rolled oats and reduce heat to low.

3. Cook for 5-7 minutes, stirring occasionally, until oats are soft and creamy.

4. Add diced apple and cinnamon to the oatmeal.

5. Cook for an additional 2-3 minutes until the apple is softened.

6. Remove from heat and stir in honey if desired.

7. Transfer to a bowl and serve warm.

Recipe 5: Vegetable Omelette

Ingredients:

- 2 eggs
- 1/4 cup chopped bell peppers (any color)
- 1/4 cup chopped tomatoes
- 1/4 cup chopped spinach
- Salt and pepper to taste
- 1 teaspoon olive oil

Instructions:

1. In a bowl, beat the eggs with salt and pepper.
2. Heat olive oil in a non-stick skillet over medium heat.
3. Add bell peppers, tomatoes, and spinach to the skillet.
4. Cook for 2-3 minutes until vegetables are softened.

5. Pour the beaten eggs over the vegetables in the skillet.

6. Cook for 2-3 minutes until the eggs are set.

7. Fold the omelette in half and transfer to a plate.

8. Serve hot with whole grain toast or bread.

Recipe 6: Baked Oatmeal Cups

Ingredients:

- 1 cup rolled oats
- 1/2 teaspoon baking powder
- 1/2 teaspoon cinnamon
- 1/4 teaspoon salt
- 1/2 cup milk of choice
- 1/4 cup maple syrup
- 1 egg
- 1 teaspoon vanilla extract
- 1/2 cup blueberries (fresh or frozen)

Instructions:

1. Preheat the oven to 350°F (175°C). Grease a muffin tin or line with paper liners.

2. In a large bowl, combine rolled oats, baking powder, cinnamon, and salt.

3. In another bowl, whisk together milk, maple syrup, egg, and vanilla extract.

4. Pour the wet ingredients into the dry ingredients and stir until well combined.

5. Gently fold in the blueberries.

6. Divide the oatmeal mixture evenly among the muffin cups.

7. Bake for 20-25 minutes until set and lightly golden on top.

8. Allow the oatmeal cups to cool slightly before serving.

Recipe 7: Quinoa Breakfast Bowl

Ingredients:

- 1/2 cup cooked quinoa
- 1/2 banana, sliced
- 1/4 cup mixed berries (strawberries, blueberries, raspberries)
- 1 tablespoon almond butter
- 1 tablespoon honey (optional)
- 1/4 teaspoon cinnamon

Instructions:

1. In a bowl, layer cooked quinoa, sliced banana, and mixed berries.
2. Drizzle almond butter and honey over the top.
3. Sprinkle with cinnamon.
4. Stir well to combine before enjoying this nutritious and filling breakfast bowl.

Recipe 8: Creamy Coconut Chia Pudding

Ingredients:

- 1/4 cup chia seeds
- 1 cup coconut milk (unsweetened)
- 1 tablespoon maple syrup
- 1/2 teaspoon vanilla extract
- Fresh fruit for topping (optional)
-

Instructions:

1. In a bowl, whisk together chia seeds, coconut milk, maple syrup, and vanilla extract.
2. Cover and refrigerate for at least 2 hours or overnight, stirring occasionally.
3. Once the chia pudding has thickened, divide it into serving bowls.
4. Top with fresh fruit if desired before serving.

Recipe 9: Classic Peanut Butter Toast

Ingredients:

- 1 slice whole grain bread
- 1 tablespoon peanut butter
- 1/2 banana, sliced
- Drizzle of honey (optional)

Instructions:

1. Toast the whole grain bread until golden brown.
2. Spread peanut butter evenly over the toast.
3. Arrange banana slices on top.
4. Drizzle with honey if desired.
5. Serve immediately for a quick and satisfying breakfast option.

Recipe 10: Apple Cinnamon Baked Oatmeal

Ingredients:

- 1/2 cup rolled oats
- 1/2 apple, diced
- 1/2 teaspoon cinnamon
- 1 tablespoon maple syrup
- 1/2 cup almond milk (unsweetened)
- 1 tablespoon chopped nuts (optional)

Instructions:

1. Preheat the oven to 350°F (175°C). Grease a small baking dish.
2. In a bowl, combine rolled oats, diced apple, cinnamon, maple syrup, and almond milk.
3. Pour the mixture into the prepared baking dish.
4. Bake for 25-30 minutes until the oatmeal is set and lightly browned on top.
5. Remove from the oven and let it cool slightly before serving.
6. Sprinkle with chopped nuts if desired before serving.

Recipe 11: Spinach and Feta Omelette

Ingredients:

- 2 eggs
- 1/4 cup fresh spinach, chopped
- 2 tablespoons crumbled feta cheese
- Salt and pepper to taste
- 1 teaspoon olive oil

Instructions:

1. In a nonstick skillet, warm the olive oil over medium heat.
2. Add the chopped spinach to the skillet and cook for 1-2 minutes until wilted.
3. Pour the whisked eggs into the skillet over the spinach.
4. Sprinkle the crumbled feta cheese evenly over the eggs.

5. Cook for 2-3 minutes until the eggs are set and the cheese is melted.

6. Carefully fold the omelette in half and transfer to a plate.

7. Serve hot with a side of whole grain toast or a slice of breakfast bread.

Recipe 12: Blueberry Almond Smoothie Bowl

Ingredients:

- 1/2 cup frozen blueberries
- 1/2 banana
- 1/4 cup Greek yogurt (unsweetened)
- 1 tablespoon almond butter
- 1/4 cup almond milk (unsweetened)
- Toppings: sliced almonds, fresh blueberries, granola

Instructions:

1. In a blender, combine frozen blueberries, banana, Greek yogurt, almond butter, and almond milk.
2. Blend until smooth and creamy.
3. Pour the smoothie into a bowl.
4. Top with sliced almonds, fresh blueberries, and granola.
5. Enjoy this nutritious and satisfying smoothie bowl for a hearty breakfast.

Recipe 13: Apple Cinnamon Breakfast Quinoa

Ingredients:

- 1/2 cup cooked quinoa
- 1/2 apple, diced
- 1/4 teaspoon cinnamon
- 1 tablespoon chopped walnuts
- 1 tablespoon maple syrup

Instructions:

1. In a bowl, combine cooked quinoa, diced apple, cinnamon, chopped walnuts, and maple syrup.
2. Stir until well mixed.
3. Microwave for 1-2 minutes until warm.
4. Serve immediately for a cozy and nutritious breakfast option.

Recipe 14: Peanut Butter Banana Breakfast Smoothie

Ingredients:

- 1/2 banana
- 1 tablespoon peanut butter
- 1/4 cup rolled oats
- 1/2 cup almond milk (unsweetened)
- 1/4 teaspoon vanilla extract
- Ice cubes

Instructions:

1. Peel and slice the banana.
2. In a blender, combine banana slices, peanut butter, rolled oats, almond milk, vanilla extract, and ice cubes.
3. Blend until smooth and creamy.
4. Pour into a glass and enjoy this protein-packed smoothie for breakfast.

Recipe 15: Chia Seed Breakfast Pudding

Ingredients:

- 2 tablespoons chia seeds
- 1/2 cup almond milk (unsweetened)
- 1/4 teaspoon vanilla extract
- 1 tablespoon maple syrup
- Fresh fruit for topping (optional)

Instructions:

1. In a bowl, combine chia seeds, almond milk, vanilla extract, and maple syrup.

2. Stir well to combine.

3. Cover and refrigerate for at least 2 hours or overnight, allowing the chia seeds to absorb the liquid and thicken.

4. Once the pudding has set, transfer it to a serving bowl.

5. Top with fresh fruit if desired before serving. Enjoy this nutritious and filling breakfast pudding.

Chapter 4

SOOTHING SOUPS AND SALADS

Recipe 1: Chicken and Vegetable Broth Soup

Ingredients:

- 1 cup low-sodium chicken broth
- 1/2 cup cooked chicken breast, shredded
- 1/4 cup carrots, diced
- 1/4 cup celery, diced
- 1/4 cup onion, chopped
- Salt and pepper to taste
- Fresh parsley for garnish

Instructions:

1. In a small pot, bring the chicken broth to a simmer over medium heat.

2. Add diced carrots, celery, and onion to the broth.

3. Cook for 5-7 minutes until the vegetables are tender.

4. Stir in shredded chicken breast and simmer for an additional 2-3 minutes.

5. Season with salt and pepper to taste.

6. Garnish with fresh parsley before serving.

Recipe 2: Lentil and Vegetable Soup

Ingredients:

- 1/2 cup dried lentils, rinsed
- 1 cup vegetable broth
- 1/4 cup carrots, diced
- 1/4 cup celery, diced
- 1/4 cup onion, chopped
- 1 clove garlic, minced
- 1/2 teaspoon cumin
- Salt and pepper to taste
- Fresh parsley for garnish

Instructions:

1. In a pot, combine lentils and vegetable broth.
2. Bring to a boil, then reduce heat to low and simmer for 20-25 minutes until lentils are tender.

3. In a separate pan, sauté carrots, celery, onion, and garlic until softened.

4. Add the sautéed vegetables to the pot of lentils.

5. Season with cumin, salt, and pepper to taste.

6. Simmer for an additional 10 minutes to allow flavors to meld.

7. Garnish with fresh parsley before serving.

Recipe 3: Creamy Butternut Squash Soup

- Ingredients:
- 1 cup butternut squash, cubed
- 1/2 cup low-sodium vegetable broth
- 1/4 cup coconut milk (unsweetened)
- 1/4 teaspoon cinnamon
- Pinch of nutmeg
- Salt and pepper to taste

Instructions:

1. Steam or roast the butternut squash until tender.
2. In a blender, combine cooked butternut squash, vegetable broth, coconut milk, cinnamon, and nutmeg.
3. Blend until smooth and creamy.
4. Transfer the mixture to a pot and heat over medium heat until warmed through.
5. Season with salt and pepper to taste.

Recipe 4: Creamy Cauliflower Soup

Ingredients:

- 1 cup cauliflower florets
- 1/2 cup low-sodium vegetable broth
- 1/4 cup unsweetened almond milk
- 1 clove garlic, minced
- 1/4 teaspoon thyme
- Salt and pepper to taste
- Fresh chives for garnish

Instructions:

1. Steam or boil cauliflower until tender.
2. In a blender, combine cooked cauliflower, vegetable broth, almond milk, minced garlic, and thyme.
3. Blend until smooth and creamy.
4. Transfer the mixture to a pot and heat over medium heat until warmed through.
5. Season with salt and pepper to taste.
6. Serve hot, garnished with fresh chives.

Recipe 5: Tomato and Basil Salad

Ingredients:

- 1 medium tomato, sliced
- 1/4 cup cucumber, sliced
- 2-3 fresh basil leaves, torn
- 1 tablespoon balsamic vinegar
- 1 teaspoon olive oil
- Salt and pepper to taste

Instructions:

1. Arrange tomato and cucumber slices on a plate.
2. Sprinkle torn basil leaves over the top.
3. Drizzle with balsamic vinegar and olive oil.
4. Season with salt and pepper to taste.
5. Serve immediately as a refreshing salad option.

Recipe 6: Greek Salad

Ingredients:

- 1/2 cucumber, diced
- 1/2 tomato, diced
- 1/4 cup red onion, thinly sliced
- 1/4 cup Kalamata olives, pitted
- 2 tablespoons crumbled feta cheese
- 1 tablespoon extra virgin olive oil
- 1 tablespoon lemon juice
- 1 teaspoon dried oregano
- Salt and pepper to taste

Instructions:

1. In a bowl, combine diced cucumber, tomato, red onion, and Kalamata olives.
2. Crumble feta cheese over the top.
3. Drizzle with olive oil and lemon juice.
4. Sprinkle with dried oregano, salt, and pepper.
5. Toss gently to combine.
6. Serve immediately as a flavorful and satisfying salad.

Recipe 7: Avocado and Chickpea Salad

Ingredients:

- 1/2 avocado, diced
- 1/4 cup canned chickpeas, rinsed and drained
- 1/4 cup cherry tomatoes, halved
- 1/4 cup cucumber, diced
- 1 tablespoon red onion, finely chopped
- 1 tablespoon fresh cilantro, chopped
- 1 tablespoon lime juice
- Salt and pepper to taste

1. **Instructions:**
2. In a bowl, combine diced avocado, chick
3. peas, cherry tomatoes, cucumber, red onion, and cilantro.
4. Drizzle with lime juice.

5. Season with salt and pepper to taste.

6. Gently toss to combine.

7. Serve immediately as a nutritious and satisfying salad option.

Recipe 8: Roasted Vegetable Salad

Ingredients:

- 1 cup mixed vegetables (such as bell peppers, zucchini, eggplant)
- 1 tablespoon olive oil
- 1/2 teaspoon Italian seasoning
- Salt and pepper to taste
- 2 cups mixed salad greens
- 1 tablespoon balsamic vinegar

Instructions:

1. Preheat the oven to 400°F (200°C).
2. Cut the mixed vegetables into bite-sized pieces.
3. Toss the vegetables with olive oil, Italian seasoning, salt, and pepper.
4. Arrange the veggies on a baking sheet in a single layer.

5. Roast in the preheated oven for 20-25 minutes until tender and lightly browned.

6. In a bowl, toss mixed salad greens with balsamic vinegar.

7. Arrange roasted vegetables on top of the salad greens.

8. Serve immediately as a hearty and flavorful salad.

Recipe 9: Quinoa and Kale Salad

Ingredients:

- 1/2 cup cooked quinoa
- 1 cup kale leaves, chopped
- 1/4 cup cherry tomatoes, halved
- 1/4 cup cucumber, diced
- 1/4 cup red bell pepper, diced
- 2 tablespoons feta cheese, crumbled
- 1 tablespoon extra virgin olive oil
- 1 tablespoon lemon juice
- Salt and pepper to taste

Instructions:

1. In a bowl, combine cooked quinoa, chopped kale leaves, cherry tomatoes, cucumber, red bell pepper, and crumbled feta cheese.
2. Drizzle with olive oil and lemon juice.
3. Season with salt and pepper to taste.
4. Toss gently to combine.
5. Serve immediately as a nutritious and satisfying salad option.

Recipe 10: Spinach and Strawberry Salad

Ingredients:

- 1 cup baby spinach leaves
- 1/2 cup strawberries, sliced
- 1/4 cup red onion, thinly sliced
- 2 tablespoons sliced almonds
- 1 tablespoon balsamic vinegar
- 1 teaspoon honey
- Salt and pepper to taste

Instructions:

1. In a bowl, combine baby spinach leaves, sliced strawberries, red onion, and sliced almonds.
2. In a small jar, combine balsamic vinegar and honey. Shake well to combine.
3. Drizzle the dressing over the salad.

4. Season with salt and pepper to taste.

5. Toss gently to combine.

6. Serve immediately as a refreshing and flavorful salad option.

Recipe 11: Creamy Carrot Ginger Soup

Ingredients:

- 1 cup carrots, chopped
- 1/2 cup potatoes, diced
- 1 tablespoon fresh ginger, minced
- 2 cups low-sodium vegetable broth
- 1/4 cup coconut milk (unsweetened)
- Salt and pepper to taste
- Fresh cilantro for garnish

Instructions:

1. In a pot, combine chopped carrots, diced potatoes, minced ginger, and vegetable broth.
2. Bring to a boil, then reduce heat and simmer for 20-25 minutes until vegetables are tender.
3. Puree the soup using an immersion blender until it's smooth.

4. Stir in coconut milk and season with salt and pepper to taste.

5. Simmer for an additional 5 minutes.

6. Serve hot, garnished with fresh cilantro.

Recipe 12: Creamy Mushroom Soup

Ingredients:

- 1 cup mushrooms, sliced
- 1/4 cup onion, chopped
- 1 clove garlic, minced
- 2 cups low-sodium vegetable broth
- 1/4 cup unsweetened almond milk
- 1 tablespoon olive oil
- Salt and pepper to taste
- Fresh parsley for garnish

1. Instructions:

1. In a pot, heat olive oil over medium heat.
2. Add sliced mushrooms, chopped onion, and minced garlic. Cook until vegetables are softened.

3. Pour in vegetable broth and bring to a simmer. Cook for 10-15 minutes.

4. Puree the soup using an immersion blender until it's smooth..

5. Stir in almond milk and season with salt and pepper to taste.

6. Simmer for an additional 5 minutes.

7. Serve hot, garnished with fresh parsley.

Recipe 13: Cucumber Tomato Salad

Ingredients:

- 1 cucumber, sliced
- 1 tomato, sliced
- 2 tablespoons red onion, thinly sliced
- 1 tablespoon fresh dill, chopped
- 1 tablespoon lemon juice
- 1 tablespoon extra virgin olive oil
- Salt and pepper to taste

Instructions:

1. In a bowl, combine sliced cucumber, tomato, red onion, and chopped dill.
2. Drizzle with lemon juice and olive oil.
3. Season with salt and pepper to taste.
4. Toss gently to combine.
5. Serve immediately as a refreshing and light salad option.

Recipe 14: Spinach and Quinoa Salad

Ingredients:

- 1 cup cooked quinoa
- 1 cup baby spinach leaves
- 1/4 cup cherry tomatoes, halved
- 2 tablespoons crumbled feta cheese
- 1 tablespoon balsamic vinegar
- 1 tablespoon extra virgin olive oil
- Salt and pepper to taste

Instructions:

1. In a bowl, combine cooked quinoa, baby spinach leaves, cherry tomatoes, and crumbled feta cheese.
2. Drizzle with balsamic vinegar and olive oil.
3. Season with salt and pepper to taste.
4. Toss gently to combine.
5. Serve immediately as a nutritious and satisfying salad option.

Recipe 15: Watermelon Feta Salad

Ingredients:

- 1 cup watermelon, diced
- 2 tablespoons crumbled feta cheese
- 1 tablespoon fresh mint leaves, chopped
- 1 tablespoon balsamic glaze
- Salt and pepper to taste

Instructions:

1. In a bowl, combine diced watermelon and crumbled feta cheese.
2. Sprinkle with chopped fresh mint leaves.
3. Drizzle with balsamic glaze.
4. Season with salt and pepper to taste.
5. Toss gently to combine.
6. Serve immediately as a refreshing and flavorful salad option.

Chapter 5

Main Course Meals

Recipe 1: Lemon Herb Roasted Chicken Breast

Ingredients:

- 1 small chicken breast
- 1 tablespoon olive oil
- 1/2 lemon, juiced
- 1 teaspoon dried thyme
- 1 teaspoon dried rosemary
- Salt and pepper to taste

Instructions:

1. Turn the oven on to 375°F, or 190°C.
2. Combine the olive oil, lemon juice, rosemary, thyme, salt, and pepper in a small bowl.
3. Transfer the chicken breast to a baking dish and cover it with the mixture.
4. Bake the chicken for 25 to 30 minutes, or until it's golden brown and cooked through.
5. Present heated beside a portion of steaming veggies.

Recipe 2: Garlic Butter Shrimp

Ingredients:

- 6-8 large shrimp, peeled and deveined
- 1 tablespoon butter
- 1 clove garlic, minced
- 1/2 teaspoon paprika
- Salt and pepper to taste
- Fresh parsley for garnish

Instructions:

1. Heat butter in a skillet over medium heat.
2. Add minced garlic and cook for 1-2 minutes until fragrant.
3. Add shrimp to the skillet and sprinkle with paprika, salt, and pepper.
4. Cook shrimp for 2-3 minutes on each side until pink and cooked through.
5. Garnish with fresh parsley before serving.

Recipe 3: Quinoa Stuffed Bell Peppers

Ingredients:

- 1 bell pepper, halved and seeds removed
- 1/4 cup cooked quinoa
- 1/4 cup black beans, drained and rinsed
- 1/4 cup corn kernels
- 1/4 cup diced tomatoes
- 1/4 teaspoon cumin
- 1/4 teaspoon chili powder
- Salt and pepper to taste
- 2 tablespoons shredded cheese (optional)

1. **Instructions:**

1. Preheat the oven to 375°F (190°C).
2. In a bowl, mix together cooked quinoa, black beans, corn kernels, diced tomatoes, cumin, chili powder, salt, and pepper.

3. Stuff the bell pepper halves with the quinoa mixture.

4. Place stuffed bell peppers on a baking sheet lined with parchment paper.

5. If desired, sprinkle shredded cheese on top.

6. Bake for 20-25 minutes until the bell peppers are tender.

7. Serve hot as a satisfying vegetarian main dish.

Recipe 4: Lentil and Vegetable Stir-Fry

Ingredients:

- 1/2 cup cooked lentils
- 1/2 cup mixed vegetables (bell peppers, zucchini, mushrooms)
- 1 tablespoon olive oil
- 1 clove garlic, minced
- 1 teaspoon ginger, minced
- 1 tablespoon soy sauce (low-sodium)
- Cooked quinoa for serving

Instructions:

1. Heat olive oil in a skillet over medium heat.
2. Add minced garlic and minced ginger to the skillet. Cook until fragrant.
3. Add mixed vegetables to the skillet and stir-fry for 3-4 minutes until tender-crisp.
4. Stir in cooked lentils and soy sauce. Cook for an additional 2-3 minutes.
5. Serve hot over cooked quinoa.

Recipe 5: Slow-Cooker Vegetable Soup

Ingredients:

- 1/2 cup chopped vegetables (carrots, celery, onions)
- 1/4 cup diced tomatoes
- 1/4 cup cooked beans (kidney beans, black beans)
- 2 cups low-sodium vegetable broth
- 1/2 teaspoon dried thyme
- 1/2 teaspoon dried rosemary
- Salt and pepper to taste

Instructions:

1. In a slow cooker, combine chopped vegetables, diced tomatoes, cooked beans, vegetable broth, thyme, rosemary, salt, and pepper.
2. Stir well to combine.
3. Cook on low for 6-8 hours or on high for 3-4 hours until vegetables are tender.
4. Serve hot as a comforting and nutritious meal.

Recipe 6: Turkey and Vegetable Stir-Fry

Ingredients:

- 1/2 cup cooked turkey breast, sliced
- 1/2 cup mixed vegetables (bell peppers, broccoli, carrots)
- 1 tablespoon olive oil
- 1 clove garlic, minced
- 1 tablespoon low-sodium soy sauce
- Cooked brown rice for serving

Instructions:

1. Heat olive oil in a skillet over medium heat.
2. Add minced garlic to the skillet and cook until fragrant.
3. Add sliced turkey breast and mixed vegetables. Stir-fry for 4-5 minutes until vegetables are tender.
4. Pour soy sauce over the mixture and stir to combine.
5. Serve hot over cooked brown rice.

Recipe 7: Lemon Garlic Herb Tilapia

Ingredients:

- 1 tilapia fillet
- 1 tablespoon olive oil
- 1/2 lemon, juiced
- 1 clove garlic, minced
- 1/2 teaspoon dried parsley
- Salt and pepper to taste

Instructions:

1. Preheat the oven to 375°F (190°C).
2. Place the tilapia fillet on a piece of aluminum foil.
3. In a small bowl, mix together olive oil, lemon juice, minced garlic, dried parsley, salt, and pepper.
4. Pour the mixture over the tilapia fillet.

5. Wrap the foil around the tilapia to form a packet.

6. Bake for 15-20 minutes until the fish is cooked through and flakes easily with a fork.

7. Serve hot with a side of steamed vegetables.

Recipe 8: Vegetable Stir-Fry with Tofu

Ingredients:

- 1/2 cup tofu, cubed
- 1/2 cup mixed vegetables (bell peppers, broccoli, carrots, snap peas)
- 1 tablespoon low-sodium soy sauce
- 1 clove garlic, minced
- 1/2 teaspoon ginger, minced
- 1 teaspoon sesame oil
- Cooked brown rice for serving

Instructions:

1. Heat sesame oil in a skillet over medium heat.
2. Add minced garlic and minced ginger to the skillet. Cook until fragrant.
3. Add cubed tofu and mixed vegetables. Stir-fry for 4-5 minutes until vegetables are tender.
4. Pour soy sauce over the mixture and stir to combine.
5. Serve hot over cooked brown rice.

Recipe 9: Coconut Curry Shrimp

Ingredients:

- 6-8 large shrimp, peeled and deveined
- 1/4 cup coconut milk
- 1 tablespoon curry powder
- 1 clove garlic, minced
- 1/2 teaspoon ginger, minced
- Salt and pepper to taste
- Fresh cilantro for garnish

Instructions:

1. In a skillet, combine coconut milk, curry powder, minced garlic, minced ginger, salt, and pepper.
2. Heat the mixture over medium heat until simmering.
3. Add shrimp to the skillet and cook for 2-3 minutes on each side until pink and cooked through.
4. Serve hot, garnished with fresh cilantro.

Recipe 10: Vegetarian Chili

Ingredients:

- 1/2 cup cooked kidney beans
- 1/2 cup cooked black beans
- 1/4 cup diced tomatoes
- 1/4 cup diced onions
- 1/4 cup diced bell peppers
- 1/4 cup corn kernels
- 1 clove garlic, minced
- 1/2 teaspoon chili powder
- 1/4 teaspoon cumin
- Salt and pepper to taste

Instructions:

1. In a pot, combine kidney beans, black beans, diced tomatoes, onions, bell peppers, corn

kernels, minced garlic, chili powder, cumin, salt, and pepper.

2. Stir well and bring to a simmer over medium heat.

3. Cook for 20-25 minutes, stirring occasionally, until flavors are melded and vegetables are tender.

4. Serve hot with a dollop of Greek yogurt or shredded cheese, if desired.

Recipe 11: Herb-Roasted Turkey Breast

Ingredients:

- 1 small turkey breast

- 1 tablespoon olive oil

- 1 teaspoon dried thyme

- 1 teaspoon dried rosemary

- 1 teaspoon dried sage

- Salt and pepper to taste

Instructions:

1. Preheat the oven to 375°F (190°C).
2. In a small bowl, mix together olive oil, thyme, rosemary, sage, salt, and pepper.
3. Rub the mixture over the turkey breast.
4. Place the turkey breast in a baking dish.
5. Roast for 1 to 1 1/2 hours, or until the internal temperature reaches 165°F (75°C).
6. Let the turkey breast rest for 10 minutes before slicing.
7. Serve hot with your favorite side dishes.

Recipe 12: Lemon Garlic Shrimp Scampi

Ingredients:

- 6-8 large shrimp, peeled and deveined
- 1 tablespoon olive oil
- 1 clove garlic, minced
- 1/2 lemon, juiced
- 1 tablespoon chopped parsley
- Salt and pepper to taste

Instructions:

1. In a skillet, heat olive oil over medium heat.
2. Add minced garlic and cook for 1-2 minutes until fragrant.
3. Add shrimp to the skillet and cook for 2-3 minutes on each side until pink and opaque.
4. Add lemon juice and chopped parsley to the skillet. Stir to combine.
5. Season with salt and pepper to taste.
6. Serve hot over cooked pasta or with crusty bread.

Recipe 13: Lentil Shepherd's Pie

Ingredients:

- 1/2 cup cooked lentils
- 1/4 cup diced carrots
- 1/4 cup diced onions
- 1/4 cup diced celery
- 1/4 cup diced mushrooms
- 1 clove garlic, minced
- 1/2 cup vegetable broth
- 1 tablespoon tomato paste
- 1 tablespoon Worcestershire sauce (optional)
- Mashed potatoes for topping

Instructions:

1. Preheat the oven to 375°F (190°C).
2. In a skillet, sauté diced carrots, onions, celery, mushrooms, and minced garlic until softened.

3. Add cooked lentils, vegetable broth, tomato paste, and Worcestershire sauce to the skillet. Stir to combine.

4. Simmer for 10-15 minutes until the mixture thickens.

5. Transfer the lentil mixture to a baking dish.

6. Top with mashed potatoes.

7. Bake for 25-30 minutes, or until the mashed potatoes are golden brown.

8. Serve hot as a comforting and hearty meal.

Recipe 14: Vegetarian Lasagna

Ingredients:

- 3 lasagna noodles
- 1/2 cup marinara sauce
- 1/2 cup ricotta cheese
- 1/4 cup shredded mozzarella cheese
- 1/4 cup diced zucchini
- 1/4 cup diced bell peppers
- 1/4 cup diced onions
- 1 clove garlic, minced
- 1 tablespoon olive oil
- Salt and pepper to taste

Instructions:

1. Preheat the oven to 375°F (190°C).
2. Cook lasagna noodles according to package instructions.

3. In a skillet, heat olive oil over medium heat.

4. Add minced garlic, diced zucchini, bell peppers, and onions. Sauté until vegetables are softened.

5. Spread marinara sauce evenly in the bottom of a baking dish.

6. Place one layer of lasagna noodles on top of the marinara sauce.

7. Spread half of the ricotta cheese over the noodles, followed by half of the sautéed vegetables.

8. Repeat the layers with remaining noodles, ricotta cheese, and vegetables.

9. Sprinkle shredded mozzarella cheese on top.

    Cover the baking dish with foil and bake for 25-30 minutes.

10. Remove foil and bake for an additional 10 minutes, or until cheese is melted and bubbly.

11. Let cool slightly before slicing and serving.

Recipe 15: Slow-Cooker Vegetable Curry

Ingredients:

- 1/2 cup diced potatoes
- 1/2 cup diced carrots
- 1/2 cup diced bell peppers
- 1/2 cup diced onions
- 1/2 cup diced tomatoes
- 1/2 cup chickpeas (cooked or canned)
- 1/2 cup coconut milk
- 1 tablespoon curry powder
- 1 teaspoon ground turmeric
- 1 teaspoon ground cumin
- Salt and pepper to taste
- Cooked rice for serving

Instructions:

1. In a slow cooker, combine diced potatoes, carrots, bell peppers, onions, tomatoes, chickpeas, coconut milk, curry powder, turmeric, cumin, salt, and pepper.

2. Stir well to combine.

3. Cook on low for 6-8 hours or on high for 3-4 hours, until vegetables are tender.

4. Serve hot over cooked rice. Enjoy your delicious and comforting vegetable curry!

Chapter 6

SIDES AND SNACKS

Recipe 1: Garlic Herb Roasted Potatoes

Ingredients:

- 1 small potato, diced
- 1 tablespoon olive oil
- 1 clove garlic, minced
- 1/2 teaspoon dried rosemary
- 1/2 teaspoon dried thyme
- Salt and pepper to taste

Instructions:

1. Preheat the oven to 400°F (200°C) and line a baking sheet with parchment paper.
2. In a bowl, toss diced potatoes with olive oil, minced garlic, dried rosemary, dried thyme, salt, and pepper until evenly coated.
3. Spread the potatoes in a single layer on the prepared baking sheet.
4. Roast for 25-30 minutes, or until golden brown and crispy.
5. Serve hot as a flavorful side dish.

Recipe 2: Homemade Guacamole

Ingredients:

- 1 ripe avocado
- 1/4 cup diced tomatoes
- 1 tablespoon diced red onion
- 1 tablespoon chopped cilantro
- 1/2 lime, juiced
- Salt and pepper to taste
- Tortilla chips or vegetable sticks for dipping

Instructions:

1. Scoop the flesh of the avocado into a bowl and mash with a fork.
2. Add diced tomatoes, diced red onion, chopped cilantro, lime juice, salt, and pepper to the mashed avocado.
3. Stir until well combined.
4. Serve with tortilla chips or vegetable sticks for dipping.

Recipe 3: Baked Zucchini Fries

Ingredients:

- 1 small zucchini, cut into fries
- 1/4 cup breadcrumbs
- 1 tablespoon grated Parmesan cheese
- 1/2 teaspoon garlic powder
- 1/2 teaspoon dried oregano
- Salt and pepper to taste
- Cooking spray

Instructions:

1. Preheat the oven to 425°F (220°C) and line a baking sheet with parchment paper.
2. In a bowl, mix breadcrumbs, grated Parmesan cheese, garlic powder, dried oregano, salt, and pepper.
3. Dip zucchini fries into the breadcrumb mixture, pressing gently to coat.

4. Place the coated zucchini fries on the prepared baking sheet.

5. Lightly spray the zucchini fries with cooking spray.

6. Bake for 20-25 minutes, or until golden brown and crispy.

7. Serve hot with a side of marinara sauce for dipping.

Recipe 4: Cucumber Hummus Bites

Ingredients:

- 4 cucumber slices
- 2 tablespoons hummus
- 1 tablespoon diced tomatoes
- 1 tablespoon diced red onion
- 1 tablespoon chopped parsley

Instructions:

1. Place cucumber slices on a plate or serving platter.
2. Spread hummus on top of each cucumber slice.
3. Top with diced tomatoes, diced red onion, and chopped parsley.
4. Serve immediately as a refreshing and satisfying finger food.

Recipe 5: Mini Oatmeal Banana Muffins

Ingredients:

- 1 ripe banana, mashed
- 1/2 cup rolled oats
- 1/4 cup milk (dairy or plant-based)
- 1 tablespoon honey or maple syrup
- 1/2 teaspoon baking powder
- 1/4 teaspoon cinnamon
- Pinch of salt

Instructions:

1. Preheat the oven to 350°F (175°C) and grease a mini muffin tin with cooking spray.
2. In a bowl, combine mashed banana, rolled oats, milk, honey or maple syrup, baking powder, cinnamon, and salt.
3. Divide the batter evenly among the mini muffin cups.

4. Bake for 12-15 minutes, or until a toothpick inserted into the center comes out clean.

5. Let the mini muffins cool in the tin for a few minutes before transferring to a wire rack to cool completely.

6. Enjoy these heartburn-friendly baked goods as a snack or side dish.

Recipe 6: Roasted Cauliflower with Herbs

Ingredients:

- 1 cup cauliflower florets
- 1 tablespoon olive oil
- 1/2 teaspoon dried thyme
- 1/2 teaspoon dried oregano
- Salt and pepper to taste

Instructions:

1. Preheat the oven to 400°F (200°C) and line a baking sheet with parchment paper.
2. In a bowl, toss cauliflower florets with olive oil, dried thyme, dried oregano, salt, and pepper until evenly coated.
3. Spread the cauliflower in a single layer on the prepared baking sheet.
4. Roast for 20-25 minutes, or until golden brown and tender.
5. Serve hot as a flavorful and nutritious side dish.

Recipe 7: Creamy Spinach Dip

Ingredients:

- 1/2 cup Greek yogurt
- 1/4 cup chopped spinach
- 1 tablespoon grated Parmesan cheese
- 1 clove garlic, minced
- 1/2 teaspoon lemon juice
- Salt and pepper to taste
- Vegetable sticks or crackers for dipping

Instructions:

1. In a bowl, combine Greek yogurt, chopped spinach, grated Parmesan cheese, minced garlic, lemon juice, salt, and pepper.
2. Stir until well combined.
3. Serve the creamy spinach dip with vegetable sticks or crackers for dipping.
4. Enjoy this delicious and healthy snack.

Recipe 8: Quinoa Stuffed Bell Peppers

Ingredients:

- 1 bell pepper
- 1/4 cup cooked quinoa
- 2 tablespoons diced tomatoes
- 2 tablespoons diced onions
- 2 tablespoons black beans
- 1 tablespoon shredded cheese (optional)
- 1/2 teaspoon dried oregano
- Salt and pepper to taste

Instructions:

1. Preheat the oven to 375°F (190°C) and line a baking dish with parchment paper.
2. Cut the top off the bell pepper and remove the seeds and membrane.

3. In a bowl, mix together cooked quinoa, diced tomatoes, diced onions, black beans, shredded cheese (if using), dried oregano, salt, and pepper.

4. Stuff the bell pepper with the quinoa mixture.

5. Place the stuffed bell pepper in the prepared baking dish.

6. Bake for 25-30 minutes, or until the bell pepper is tender.

7. Serve hot as a satisfying side dish or snack.

Recipe 9: Baked Sweet Potato Fries

Ingredients:

- 1 small sweet potato, cut into fries
- 1 tablespoon olive oil
- 1/2 teaspoon paprika
- 1/4 teaspoon garlic powder
- Salt and pepper to taste

Instructions:

1. Preheat the oven to 425°F (220°C) and line a baking sheet with parchment paper.
2. In a bowl, toss sweet potato fries with olive oil, paprika, garlic powder, salt, and pepper until evenly coated.
3. Spread the sweet potato fries in a single layer on the prepared baking sheet.
4. Bake for 20-25 minutes, flipping halfway through, until golden brown and crispy.
5. Serve hot as a delicious and nutritious side dish or snack.

Recipe 10: Almond Butter Energy Balls

Ingredients:

- 1/2 cup rolled oats
- 1/4 cup almond butter
- 2 tablespoons honey or maple syrup
- 1 tablespoon chia seeds
- 1 tablespoon shredded coconut (optional)
- 1/4 teaspoon vanilla extract

Instructions:

1. In a bowl, mix together rolled oats, almond butter, honey or maple syrup, chia seeds, shredded coconut (if using), and vanilla extract until well combined.
2. Roll the mixture into small balls using your hands.
3. Place the energy balls on a plate or baking sheet lined with parchment paper.
4. Refrigerate for at least 30 minutes to firm up.
5. Enjoy these nutritious and energy-boosting snacks on the go.

Chapter 7

BEVERAGES AND DESSERTS

Recipe 1: Peppermint Tea

Ingredients:

- 1 peppermint tea bag
- 1 cup hot water
- Honey or lemon (optional)

Instructions:

1. Place the peppermint tea bag in a cup.
2. Pour hot water over the tea bag.
3. Let it steep for 5-7 minutes.
4. Remove the tea bag.
5. Add honey or lemon if desired.
6. Sip on this soothing tea to ease digestion and relieve heartburn.

Recipe 2: Ginger Turmeric Tea

Ingredients:

- 1 teaspoon grated fresh ginger
- 1/2 teaspoon ground turmeric
- 1 cup hot water
- Honey (optional)

Instructions:

1. Place grated ginger and ground turmeric in a cup.
2. Pour hot water over the ingredients.
3. Let it steep for 5-7 minutes.
4. Strain the tea if desired.
5. Add honey for sweetness if desired.
6. Enjoy the anti-inflammatory and digestive benefits of this comforting tea.

Recipe 3: Honey Lemon Chamomile Tea

Ingredients:

- 1 chamomile tea bag
- 1/2 lemon, juiced
- 1 teaspoon honey
- 1 cup hot water

Instructions:

1. Place the chamomile tea bag in a cup.
2. Squeeze lemon juice into the cup.
3. Add honey to taste.
4. Pour hot water over the ingredients.
5. Let it steep for 5-7 minutes.
6. Remove the tea bag.
7. Stir well and enjoy this soothing and refreshing tea.

Recipe 4: Berry Smoothie

Ingredients:

- 1/2 cup mixed berries (strawberries, blueberries, raspberries)
- 1/2 banana
- 1/2 cup plain Greek yogurt
- 1/2 cup almond milk
- 1 tablespoon honey (optional)

Instructions:

1. Combine mixed berries, banana, Greek yogurt, almond milk, and honey (if using) in a blender.
2. Blend until smooth and creamy.
3. Pour into a glass and enjoy this nutritious and refreshing smoothie.

Recipe 5: Banana Oat Cookies

Ingredients:

- 1 ripe banana, mashed
- 1/2 cup rolled oats
- 1 tablespoon almond butter
- 1 tablespoon honey
- 1/4 teaspoon cinnamon
- Pinch of salt

Instructions:

1. Preheat the oven to 350°F (175°C) and line a baking sheet with parchment paper.
2. In a bowl, mix together mashed banana, rolled oats, almond butter, honey, cinnamon, and a pinch of salt until well combined.
3. Drop spoonfuls of the mixture onto the prepared baking sheet and flatten slightly with the back of a spoon.
4. Bake for 12-15 minutes or until golden brown.
5. Allow the cookies to cool before enjoying these guilt-free treats.

Recipe 6: Coconut Chia Pudding

Ingredients:

- 2 tablespoons chia seeds
- 1/2 cup coconut milk
- 1 teaspoon honey or maple syrup
- 1/4 teaspoon vanilla extract
- Fresh fruit for topping (optional)

Instructions:

1. In a small bowl or jar, mix together chia seeds, coconut milk, honey or maple syrup, and vanilla extract.
2. Stir well to combine.
3. Cover and refrigerate for at least 2 hours or overnight, until the mixture thickens and sets.
4. Serve chilled, topped with fresh fruit if desired.

Recipe 7: Apple Cinnamon Baked Oatmeal

Ingredients:

- 1/2 cup rolled oats
- 1/2 apple, diced
- 1/2 teaspoon cinnamon
- 1/2 cup almond milk
- 1 tablespoon maple syrup
- 1 tablespoon chopped nuts (optional)

Instructions:

1. Preheat the oven to 350°F (175°C) and grease a small baking dish.

2. In a bowl, mix together rolled oats, diced apple, cinnamon, almond milk, and maple syrup.

3. Pour the mixture into the prepared baking dish.

4. Bake for 25-30 minutes, or until the oats are cooked and the top is golden brown.

5. Sprinkle with chopped nuts if desired.

6. Serve warm as a comforting and nutritious dessert or breakfast.

Recipe 8: Avocado Chocolate Mousse

Ingredients:

- 1 ripe avocado
- 2 tablespoons cocoa powder
- 2 tablespoons honey or maple syrup
- 1/4 teaspoon vanilla extract
- Pinch of salt
- Fresh berries for garnish (optional)

Instructions:

1. Scoop the flesh of the avocado into a blender or food processor.
2. Add cocoa powder, honey or maple syrup, vanilla extract, and a pinch of salt.
3. Blend until smooth and creamy, scraping down the sides as needed.
4. Transfer the mousse to serving bowls.
5. Refrigerate for at least 30 minutes to chill.
6. Garnish with fresh berries before serving if desired.

Recipe 9: Greek Yogurt Parfait

Ingredients:

- 1/2 cup plain Greek yogurt
- 1/4 cup granola
- 1/4 cup mixed berries (strawberries, blueberries, raspberries)
- 1 tablespoon honey or maple syrup (optional)

Instructions:

1. In a glass or bowl, layer Greek yogurt, granola, and mixed berries.
2. Repeat layers until ingredients are used up.
3. Drizzle with honey or maple syrup if desired.
4. Serve immediately as a delicious and satisfying dessert or snack.

Recipe 10: Baked Apples with Cinnamon

Ingredients:

- 1 apple, cored and sliced
- 1/2 teaspoon cinnamon
- 1 teaspoon honey or maple syrup
- 1 tablespoon chopped nuts (optional)

Instructions:

1. Preheat the oven to 350°F (175°C) and grease a baking dish.
2. Place apple slices in the baking dish.
3. Sprinkle with cinnamon and drizzle with honey or maple syrup.
4. Toss to coat evenly.
5. Bake for 20-25 minutes, or until the apples are tender.
6. Sprinkle with chopped nuts if desired.
7. Serve warm as a comforting and healthy dessert.

Conclusion: A Toast to a Life Well-Lived, One Bite at a Time

Arriving at the final pages, it's important to reflect on the transformative power of knowledge and self-care. The path you've undertaken through this book is not merely a quest for relief from acid reflux; it's a profound commitment to embracing a life free from the burdens of discomfort and pain.

Throughout these chapters, we've explored the intricacies of a heartburn-friendly diet, empowering you with the tools to identify and avoid trigger foods while embracing a world of delicious, nourishing alternatives. From alkaline-forming foods that neutralize stomach acid to fiber-rich options that promote healthy digestion, you now possess a wealth of culinary knowledge to guide your choices.

But our journey has transcended mere dietary modifications. We've delved into the realm of lifestyle adjustments, recognizing that true well-being is achieved through a holistic approach. By embracing practical techniques such as maintaining a healthy weight, practicing stress-reducing activities, and optimizing your sleep patterns, you've taken ownership of your overall wellness, creating a harmonious balance between mind, body, and spirit.

The recipes and strategies you've encountered within these pages are not just a collection of guidelines; they are a testament to the resilience of the human spirit and the unwavering pursuit of joy. Each meal you prepare, each mindful decision you make, is a celebration of your commitment to reclaiming the simple pleasures of life – savoring every bite without the burden of discomfort.

As you embark on this newfound path, remember that you are not alone. This book has been your companion, a trusted ally in navigating the challenges of acid reflux. But more importantly, you now belong to a community of individuals who have embraced the power of self-care and emerged victorious in their quest for a life well-lived.

Carry this knowledge with you, like a cherished heirloom, and pass it on to those who may benefit from your hard-won wisdom. Share the recipes that have brought you comfort and joy, and inspire others to embark on their own journeys towards a heartburn-free existence.

In the end, this book is not merely a collection of pages; it is a testament to the indomitable human spirit, a celebration of resilience, and a reminder that true joy can be found in the simplest of pleasures – a shared meal, a heartfelt laugh, and the knowledge that every bite is a step towards a life well-lived.

So raise a glass, or perhaps a mug of soothing herbal tea, and toast to the journey that lies ahead. A journey filled with delicious discoveries, heartwarming moments, and the unwavering belief that a life free from the discomfort of acid reflux is not only possible but within your grasp.

Bonus Chapter: Weekly Meal Planner

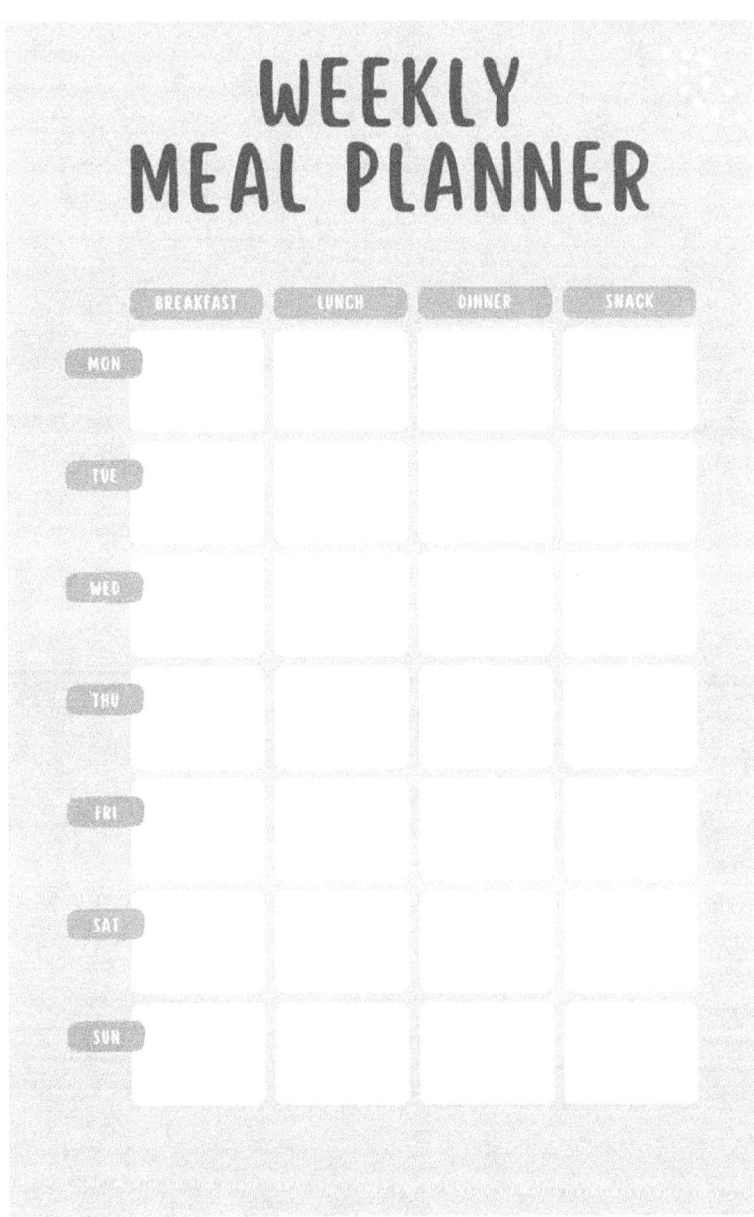

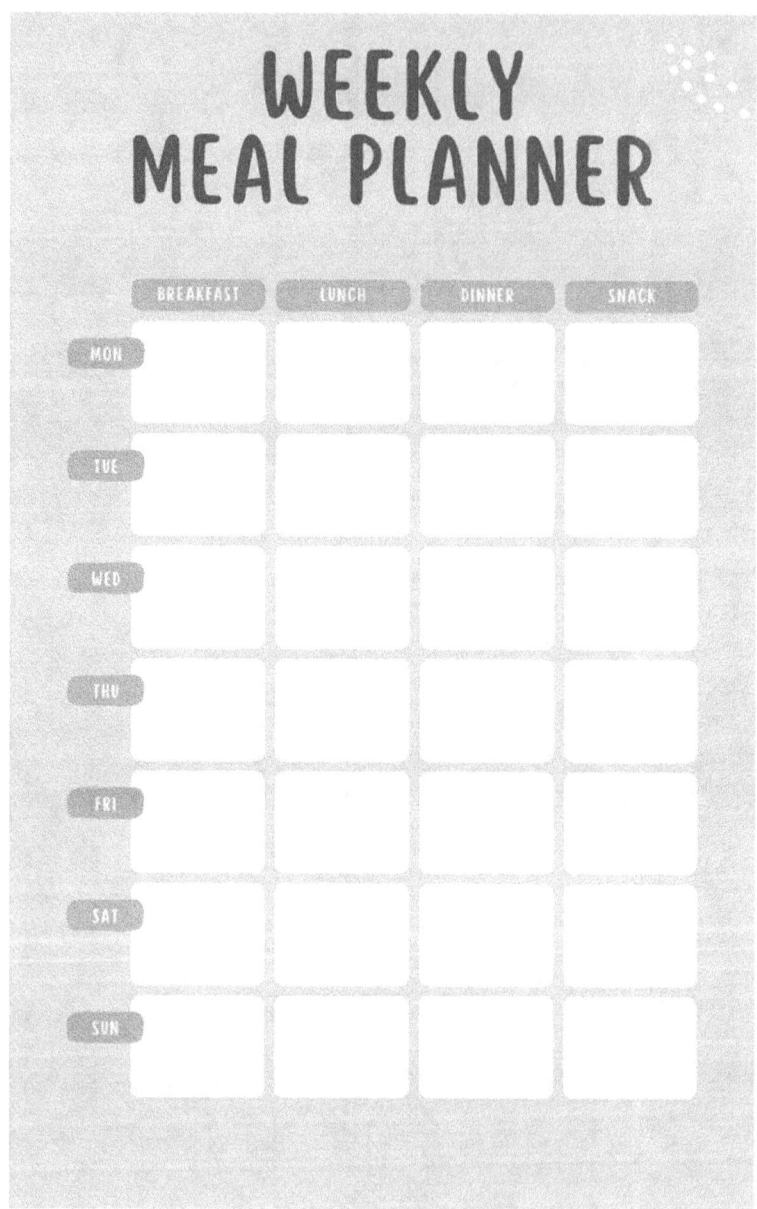

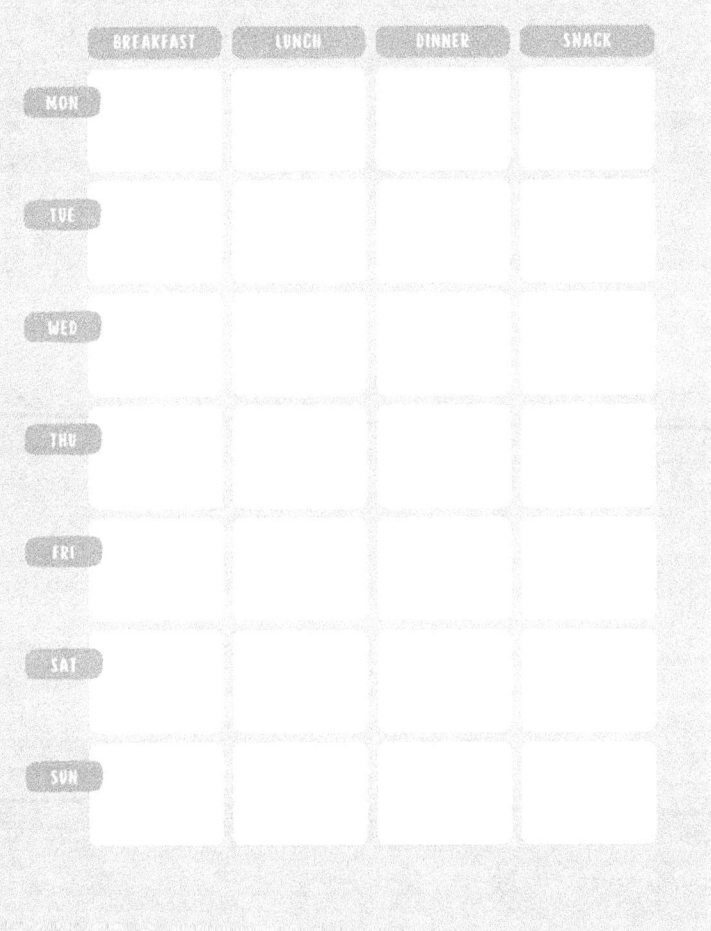

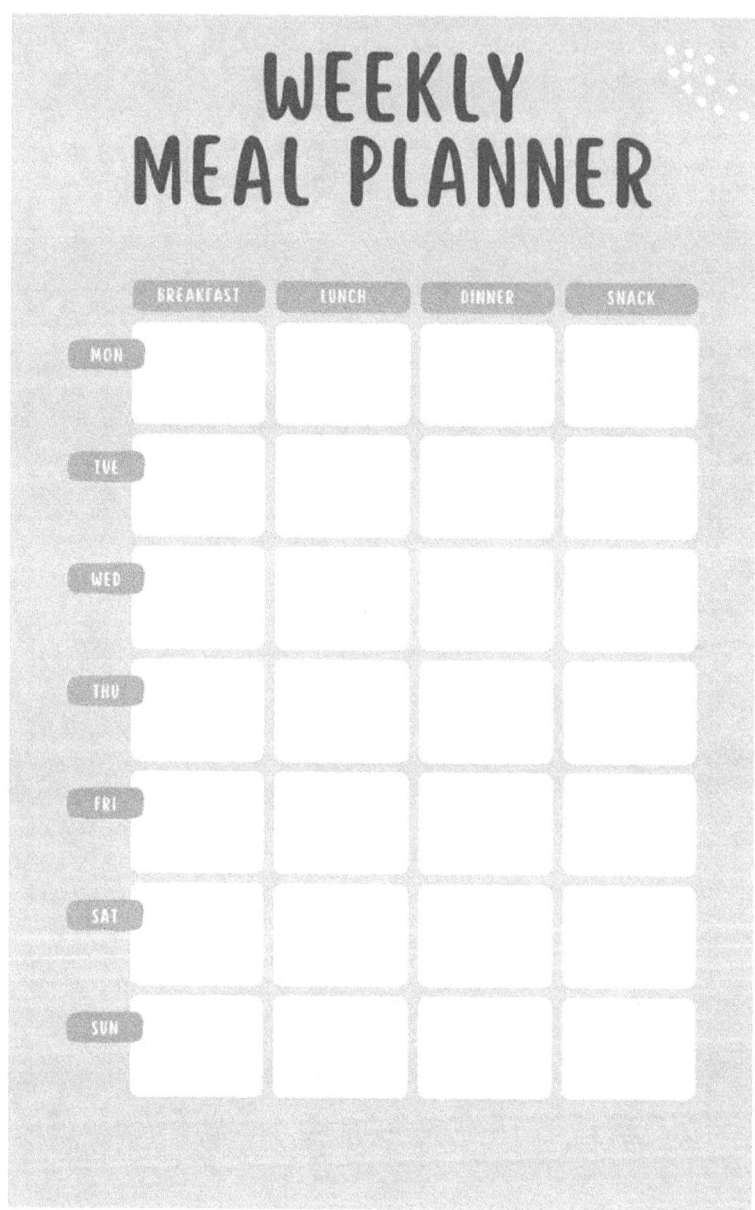

WEEKLY MEAL PLANNER

	BREAKFAST	LUNCH	DINNER	SNACK
MON				
TUE				
WED				
THU				
FRI				
SAT				
SUN				

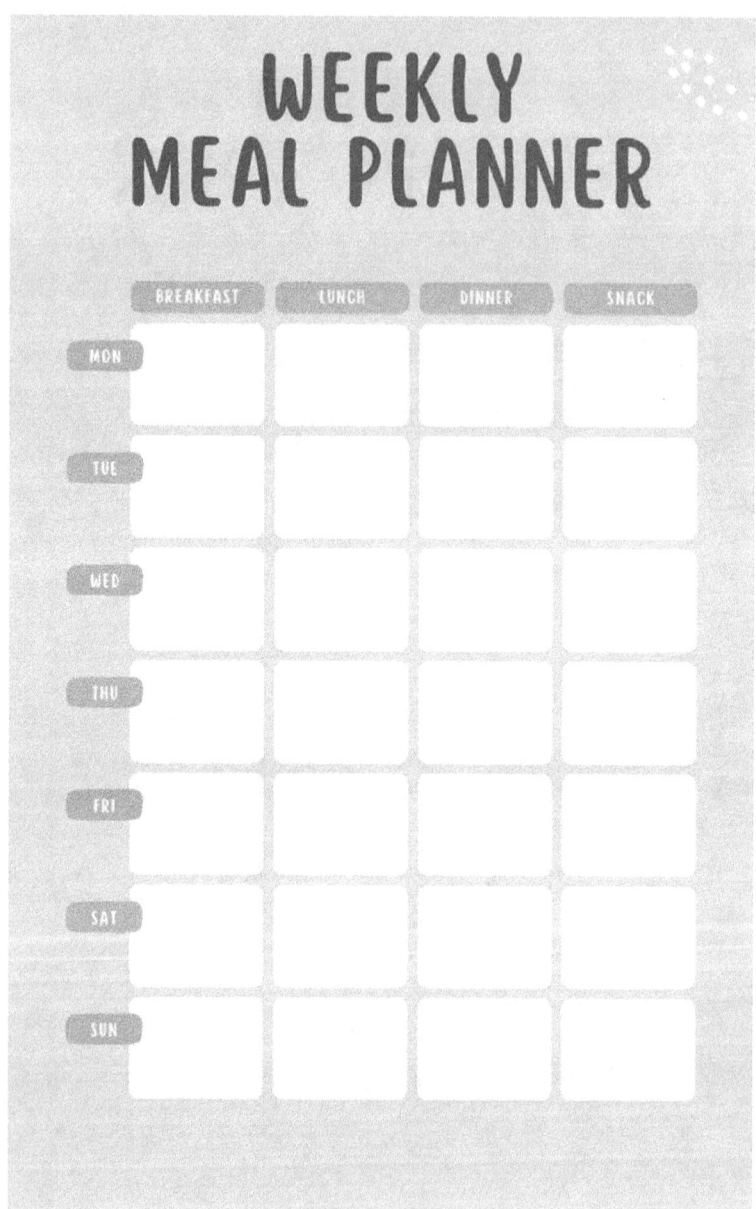

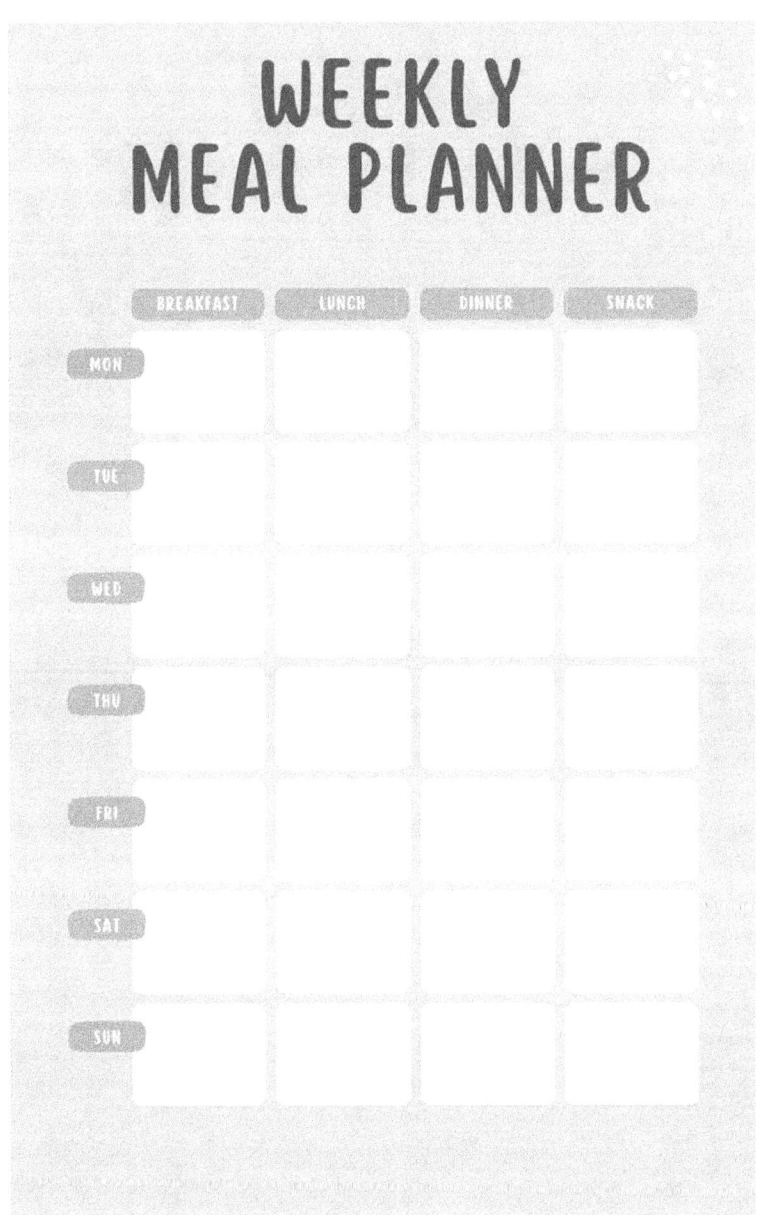

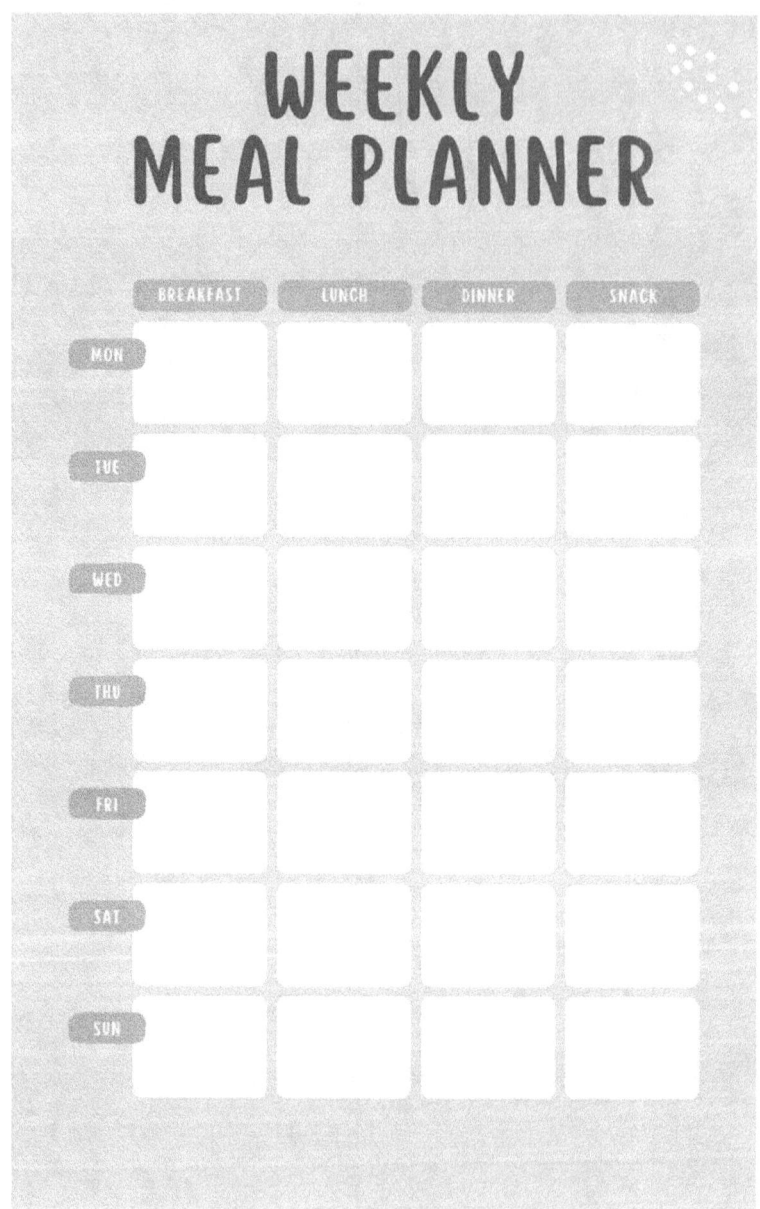

WEEKLY MEAL PLANNER

	BREAKFAST	LUNCH	DINNER	SNACK
MON				
TUE				
WED				
THU				
FRI				
SAT				
SUN				

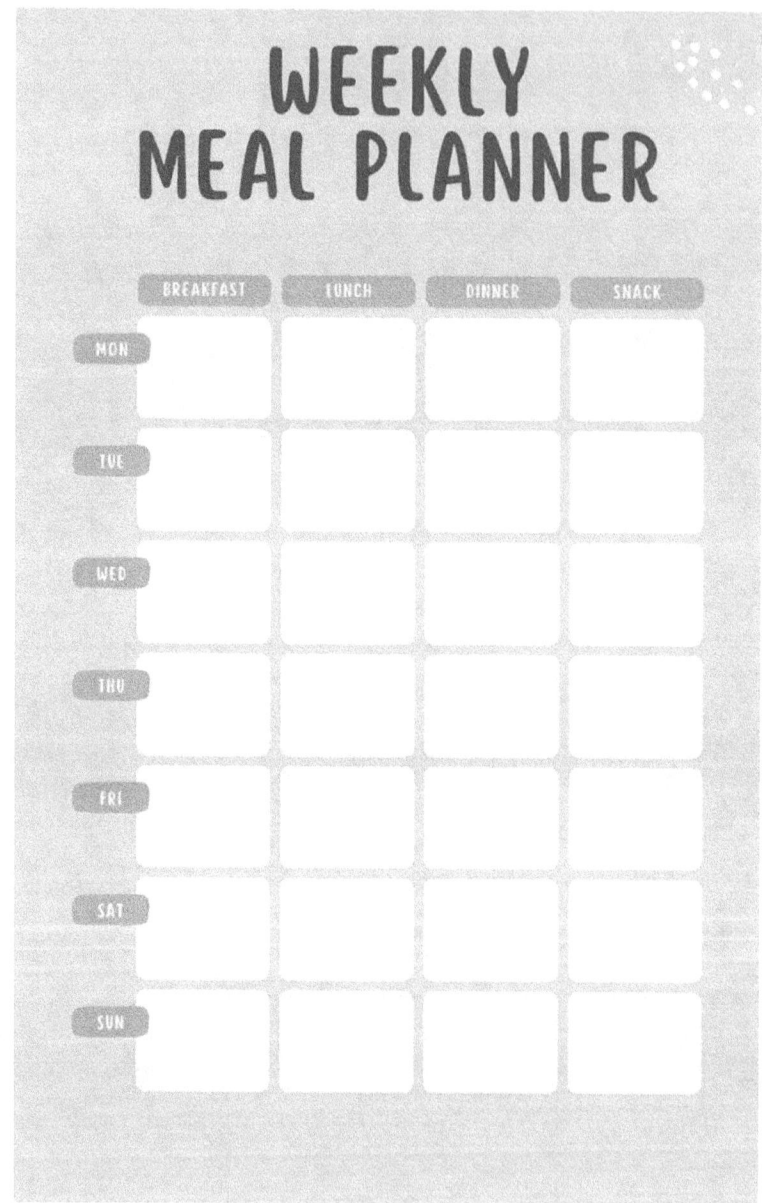

WEEKLY MEAL PLANNER

	BREAKFAST	LUNCH	DINNER	SNACK
MON				
TUE				
WED				
THU				
FRI				
SAT				
SUN				

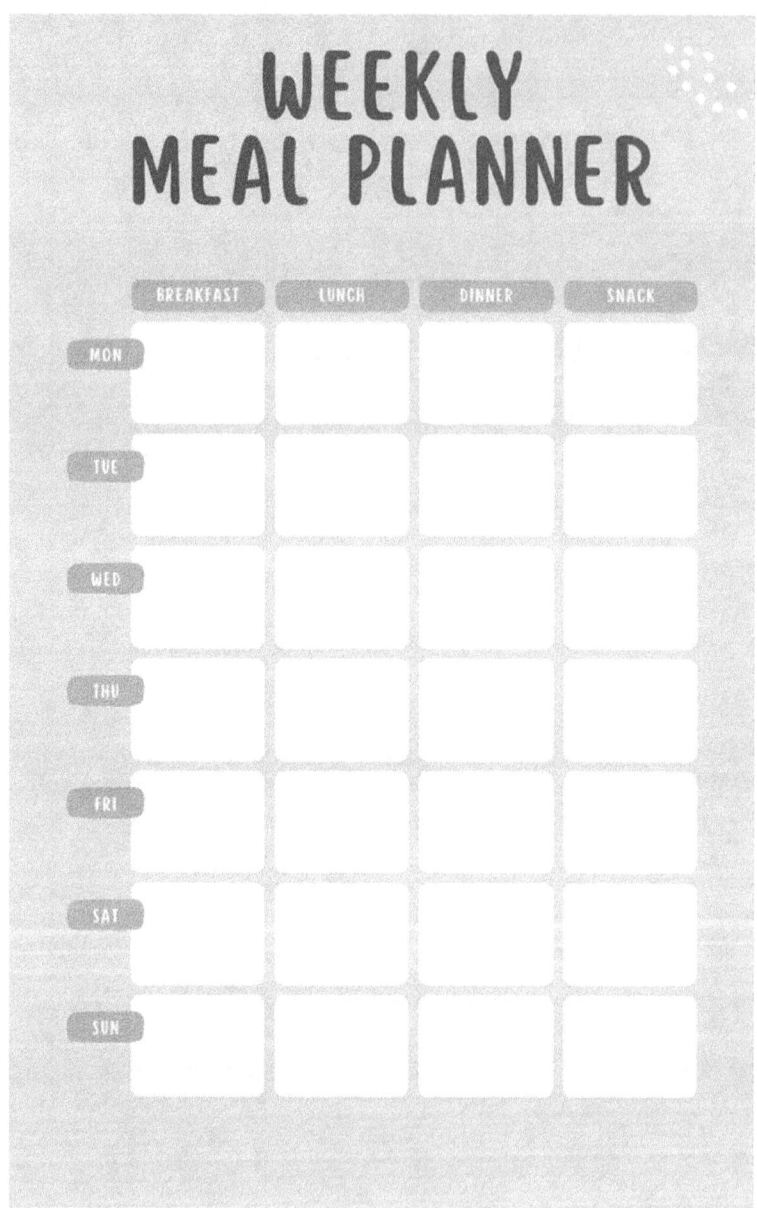

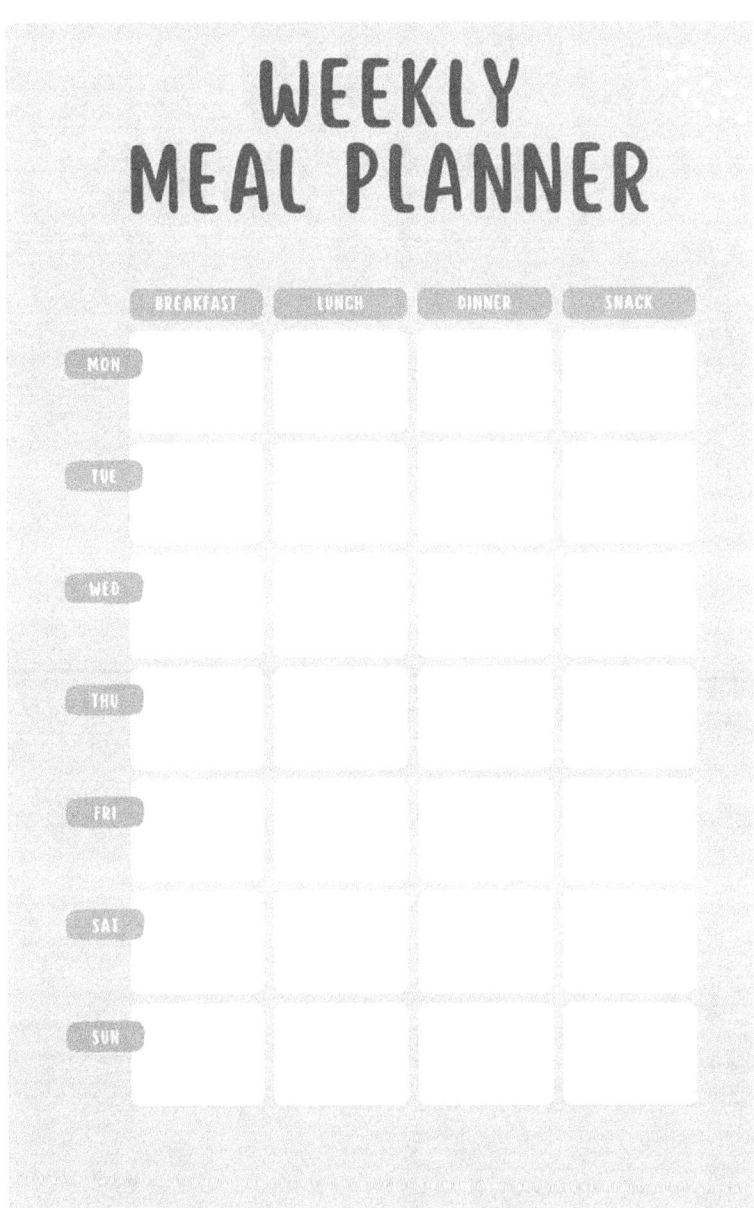

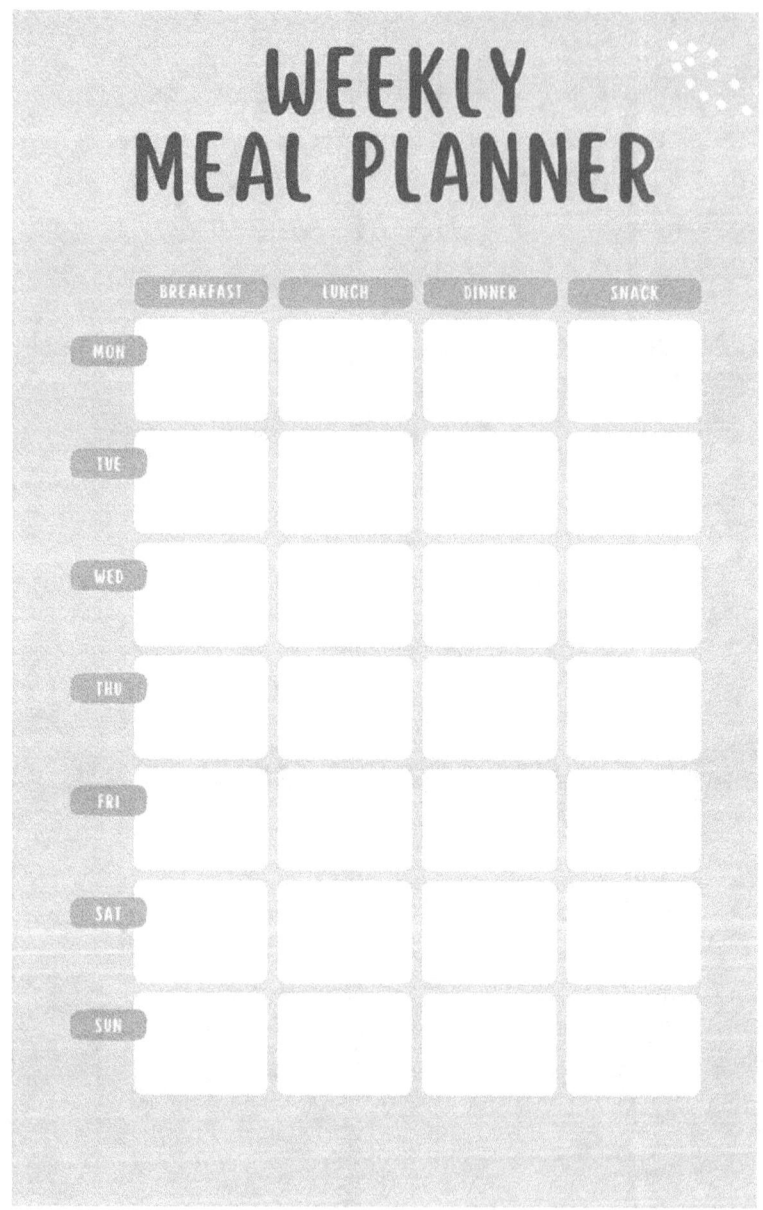

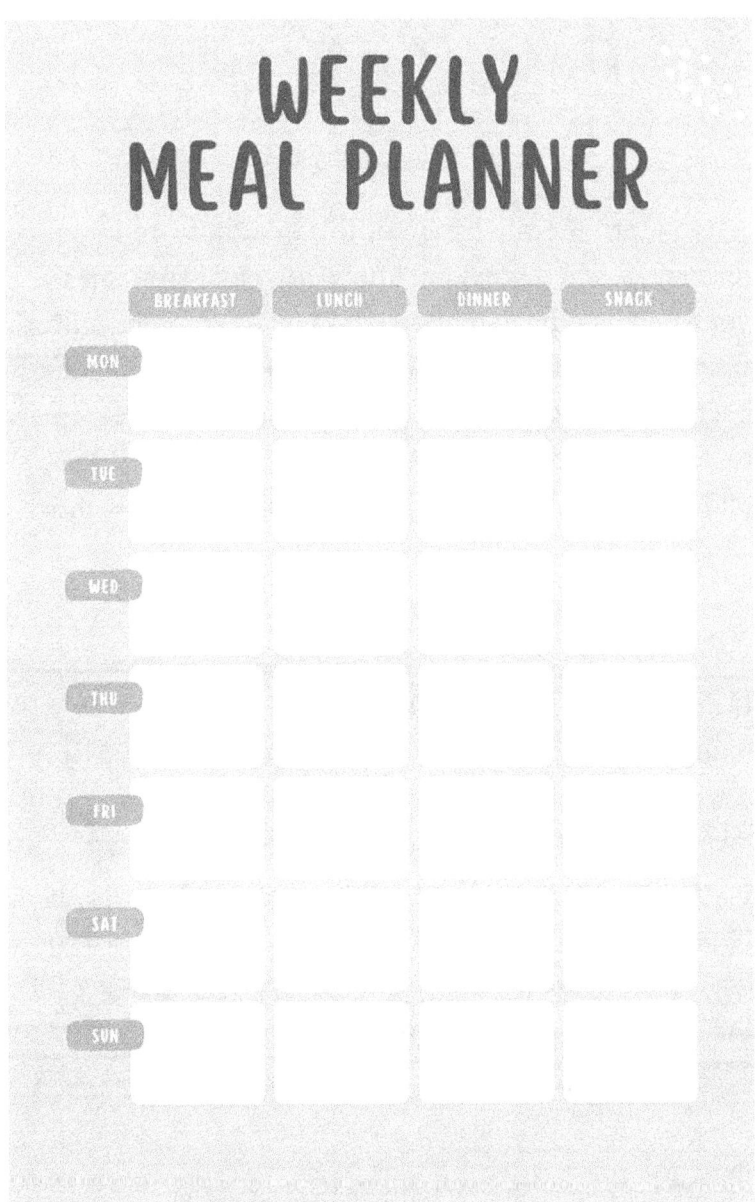

Thanks for Reading

As you turn the final page of this heartburn-relieving journey, we hope that the knowledge and strategies you've gained have empowered you to embrace a life free from the discomfort of acid reflux. This book has been a labor of love, a culmination of extensive research, personal experiences, and a deep understanding of the unique challenges faced by older adults.

If the recipes, dietary guidelines, and lifestyle modifications contained within these pages have truly resonated with you, we would be honored if you could take a moment to share your thoughts and leave a review on Amazon. Your feedback not only helps us improve and refine our approach but also serves as a beacon of hope for others who are still grappling with the challenges of acid reflux.

Please feel free to reach out to us at **drjulianaandrew@gmail.com** if you have any further questions, concerns, or simply wish to share your personal journey towards a heartburn-free life.

We are here to support you every step of the way, offering guidance, encouragement, and a listening ear.

Remember, this book is not just a collection of recipes and advice; it's a testament to the resilience of the human spirit and the unwavering belief that true joy can be found in the simplest of pleasures – a shared meal, a heartfelt laugh, and the knowledge that every bite is a step towards a life well-lived.

Thank you for embarking on this journey with us. May your days be filled with delicious discoveries, heartwarming moments, and the unwavering belief that a life free from the discomfort of acid reflux is not only possible but within your grasp.

Warmly,

Dr. Juliana Andrew

www.ingramcontent.com/pod-product-compliance
Lightning Source LLC
Chambersburg PA
CBHW070146230526
45471CB00002B/541